Weight Loss Hypnosis For Women

The Ultimate guide to the best Remedies for Women to Get Lean Quickly through Self-Hypnosis, Meditation, and Affirmations to Burn Fat and Stop Sugar Craving

Elizabeth Collins

Table of Contents

Introduction

Hypnosis is rewiring your brain to add or to change your daily routine starting from your basic instincts. This happens due to the fact that while you are in a hypnotic state you are more susceptible to suggestions by the person who put you in this state. In the case of self-hypnosis, the person who made you enter the trance of hypnotism is yourself. Thus, the only person who can give you suggestions that can change your attitude in this method is you and you alone.

Again, you must forget the misconception that hypnosis is like sleeping because if it is then it would be impossible to give autosuggestions to yourself. Try to think about it like being in a very vivid daydream where you are capable of controlling every aspect of the situation you are in. This gives you the ability to change anything that may bother and hinder you to achieve the best possible result. If you are able to pull it off properly, then the possibility of improving yourself after a constant practice of the method will just be a few steps away.

Career

People say that motivation is the key to improve in your career. But no matter how you love your career, you must admit that there are aspects in your work that you really do not like doing. Even if it is a fact that you are good in the other tasks, there is that one duty that you dread. And every time you encounter this specific chore you seem to be slowed down and thus lessening your productivity at work. This is where self-hypnosis comes into play.

The first thing you need to do is find that task you do not like. In some cases there might be multiple of them depending on your personality and how you feel about your job. Now, try to look at why you do not like that task and do simple research on how to make the job a lot simpler. You can then start conditioning yourself to use the simple method every time you do the job.

After you are able to condition your state of mind to do the task, each time you encounter it will become the trigger for your trance and thus giving you the ability to perform it better. You will not be able to tell the difference since you will not mind it at all. Your coworkers and superiors though will definitely notice the change in your work style and in your productivity.

Family

It is easy to improve in a career. But to improve your relationship with your family can be a little tricky. Yet, self-hypnosis can still reprogram you to interact with your family members better by modifying how you react to the way they act. You will have the ability to adjust your way of thinking depending on the situation. This then allows you to respond in the most positive way possible, no matter how dreadful the scenario may be.

If you are in a fight with your husband/wife, for example, the normal reaction is to flare up and face fire with fire. The problem with this approach is it usually engulfs the entire relationship which might eventually lead up to separation. Being in a hypnotic state in this instance can help you think clearly and change the impulse of saying the words without thinking through. Anger will still be there, of course, that is the healthy way. But anger now under self-hypnosis can be channeled and stop being a raging inferno, you can turn it into a steady bonfire that can help you and your partner find common ground for whatever issue you are facing. The same applies in dealing with a sibling or children. If you are able to condition your mind to think more rationally or to get into the perspective of others, then you can have better family/friends' relationships.

Health and Physical Activities

Losing weight can be the most common reason why people will use self-hypnosis in terms of health and physical activities. But this is just one part of it. Self-hypnosis can give you a lot more to improve this aspect of your life. It works the same way while working out.

Most people tend to give up their exercise program due to the exhaustion they think they can no longer take. But through self-hypnosis, you will be able to tell yourself that the exhaustion is lessened and thus allowing you to finish the entire routine. Keep in mind though that your mind must never be conditioned to forget exhaustion, it must only not mind it until the end of the exercise. Forgetting it completely might lead you to not stopping to work out until your energy is depleted. It becomes counterproductive in this case.

Having a healthy diet can also be influenced by self-hypnosis. Conditioning your mind to avoid unhealthy food can be done. Thus, hypnosis will be triggered each you are tempted to eat a meal you are conditioned to consider as unhealthy. Your eating habit then can change to benefit you to improve your overall health.

Mental, Emotional and Spiritual Needs

Since self-hypnosis deals directly in how you think, it is then no secret that it can greatly improve your mental, emotional and spiritual needs. A clear mind can give your brain the ability to have more rational thoughts. Rationality then leads to better decision making and easy absorption and retention of information you might need to improve your mental capacity. You must set your expectations, though; this does not work like magic that can turn you into a genius. The process takes time depending on how far you want to go, how much you want to achieve. Thus, the effects will only be limited by how much you are able to condition your mind.

In terms of emotional needs, self-hypnosis cannot make you feel differently in certain situations. But it can condition you to take in each scenario a little lighter and make you deal with them better. Others think that getting rid of emotion can be the best course of action if you are truly able to rewire your brain. But they seem to forget that even though rational thinking is often influenced negatively by emotion, it is still necessary for you to decide on things basing on the common ethics and aesthetics of the real world. Self-hypnosis then can channel your emotion to work in a more positive way in terms of decision making and dealing with emotional hurdles and problems.

Spiritual need on the other hand is far easier to influence when it comes to doing self-hypnosis. As a matter of fact, most people with spiritual beliefs are able to do self-hypnosis each time they practice what they believe in. A deep prayer, for instance, is a way to self-hypnotize yourself to enter the trance to feel closer to a Divine existence. Chanting and meditation done by other religions also leads and have the same goal. Even the songs during a mass or praise and worship triggers self-hypnosis depending if the person allows them to do so.

Still, the improvements can only be achieved if you condition yourself that you are ready to accept them. The willingness to put an effort must also be there. An effortless hypnosis will only create the illusion that you are improving and thus will not give you the satisfaction of achieving your goal in reality.

How hypnosis can help resolve childhood issues

Another issue that hypnosis can help you with are problems from our past. If you have had traumatic situations from your childhood days, then you may have issues in all areas of your adult life. Unresolved issues from your past can lead to anxiety and depression in your later years. Childhood trauma is dangerous because it can alter many things in the brain both psychologically and chemically.

The most vital thing to remember about trauma from your childhood is that given a harmless and caring environment in which the child's vital needs for physical safety, importance, emotional security and attention are met, the damage that trauma and abuse cause can be eased and relieved. Safe and dependable relationships are also a dynamic component in healing the effects of childhood trauma in adulthood and make an atmosphere in which the brain can safely start the process of recovery.

Pure Hypnoanalysis is the lone most effective method of treatment available in the world today, for the resolution of phobias, anxiety, depression, fears, psychological and emotional problems/symptoms and eating disorders. It is a highly advanced form of hypnoanalysis (referred to as analytical hypnotherapy or hypno-analysis). Hypnoanalysis, in its numerous forms, is practiced all over the world; this method of hypnotherapy can completely resolve the foundation of anxieties in the unconscious mind, leaving the individual free of their symptoms for life.

There is a deeper realism active at all times around us and inside us. This reality commands that we must come to this world to find happiness, and every so often that our inner child stands in our way. This is by no means intentional; however, it desires to reconcile wounds from the past or address damaging philosophies which were troubling to us as children.

So disengaging the issues that upset us from earlier in our lives we have to find a way to bond with our internal child, we then need to assist in rebuilding this part of us which will, in turn, help us to be rid of all that has been hindering us from moving on.

Connecting with your inner child may seem like something

that may be hard or impossible to do, especially since they may be a part that has long been buried. It is a fairly easy exercise to do and can even be done right now. You will need about 20 minutes to complete this exercise. Here's what you do: find a quiet spot where you won't be disturbed and find pictures of you as a child if you think it may help.

Breathe in and loosen your clothing if you have to. Inhale deeply into your abdomen and exhale, repeat until you feel yourself getting relaxed; you may close your eyes and focus on getting less tense. Feel your forehead and head relax, let your face become relaxed and relax your shoulders. Allow your body to be limp and loose while you breathe slowly. Keep breathing slowly as you let all of your tension float away.

Now slowly count from 10 to 0 in your mind and try to think of a place from your childhood. The image doesn't have to be crystal clear right now but try to focus on exactly how you remember it and keep that image in mind. Imagine yourself as a child and imagine observing younger you; think about your clothes, expression, hair, etc. In your mind go and meet yourself, introduce yourself to you.

Chapter 1: Lose Weight Fast and Naturally

Numerous individuals are uncertain about how to lose weight securely and normally. It does not support that multiple sites and notices, especially those having a place with companies that sell diet drugs or other weight-loss products, promote misinformation about losing weight.

As indicated by 2014 research, a great many people who look for tips on the most proficient method to get thinner will go over false or deluding information on weight reduction.

"Fad" diets and exercise regimens can at times be hazardous as they can keep individuals from meeting their nourishing needs.

As indicated by the Centers for Disease Control and Prevention, the most secure measure of weight to lose every week is somewhere in the range of 1 and 2 pounds. The individuals who suffer substantially more every week or attempt craze diets or projects are significantly more prone to recover weight.

1. Keeping Refreshing Bites at Home and In the Workplace

Individuals frequently pick to eat nourishments that are helpful, so it is ideal to abstain from keeping prepackaged tidbits and confections close by.

One investigation found that individuals who kept unhealthful nourishment at home thought that it was increasingly hard to keep up or lose weight.

Keeping healthful snacks at home and work can enable an individual to meet their nourishing needs and maintain a strategic distance from an abundance of sugar and salt. Great snack choices include:

- nuts with no added salt or sugar
- natural products
- prechopped vegetables
- low-fat yoghurts
- dried seaweed

2. Removing Processed Foods

Processed foods are high in sodium, fat, calories, and sugar. They frequently contain fewer supplements than entire nourishments.

As indicated by a primer research study, processed foods are substantially more likely than different food sources to prompt addictive eating practices, which will, in general, outcome in individuals indulging.

3. Eating More Protein

An eating routine high in protein can enable an individual to lose weight. A diagram of existing examination on high protein eats fewer carbs inferred that they are an effective system for forestalling or treating obesity.

The information demonstrated that higher-protein diets of 25–30 grams of protein for each feast gave enhancements in hunger, bodyweight the board, cardiometabolic hazard components, or these wellbeing results.

- fish
- beans, peas, and lentils
- white poultry
- low-fat cottage cheese
- tofu

4. Stopping Included Sugar

Sugar is not in every case simple to maintain a strategic distance from; however, disposing of handled nourishments is a positive initial step to take.

As per the National Cancer Institute, men matured 19 years and more established devour a normal of more than 19 teaspoons of included sugar a day. Ladies in a similar age bunch eat more than 14 teaspoons of added sugar a day.

A significant part of the sugar that individuals devour originates from fructose, which the liver separates and transforms into fat. After the liver converts the sugar into fat, it discharges these fat cells into the blood, which can prompt weight gain.

5. Drinking Black Coffee

Coffee may have some constructive wellbeing impacts if an individual forgoes, including sugar and fat. The writers of a survey article saw that coffee improved the body's processing of carbohydrates and fats.

A like look at featured a relationship between coffee utilization and a lower danger of diabetes and liver disease.

6. Remaining Hydrated

Water is the best liquid that an individual can drink for the day. It contains no calories and gives an abundance of health benefits.

At the point when an individual drinks water for the day, the water helps increment their digestion. Drinking water before a feast can likewise help decrease the sum that they eat.

At long last, if individuals supplant sweet refreshments with water, this will help decrease all outnumber of calories that they devour for the day.

7. Keeping Away from The Calories in Beverages

Soft drinks, natural product squeezes, and sports and caffeinated drinks regularly contain abundant sugar, which can prompt weight increase and make it progressively hard for an individual to get in shape.

Other high-calorie drinks incorporate liquor and strength espressos, like lattes, which contain milk and sugar.

Individuals can have a go at supplanting, at any rate, one of these drinks every day with water, shining water with lemon, or an herbal tea.

8. Avoiding Refined Carbohydrates

Proof in The American Journal of Clinical Nutrition recommends that refined sugars might be more harmful to the body's digestion than saturated fats.

Considering the convergence of sugar from refined starches,

the liver will make and discharge fat into the circulatory system.

To diminish weight and keep it off, an individual can eat entire grains.

Refined or simple carbohydrates incorporate the accompanying nourishments:

- white rice
- white bread
- white flour
- candies
- numerous sorts of cereal
- included sugars
- numerous sorts of pasta

Rice, bread, and pasta are, for the most part, accessible in entire grain varieties, which can help weight reduction and help shield the body from disease.

9. Fasting in Cycles

Fasting for short periods may enable an individual to get more fit. As per a recent report, irregular fasting or substitute day fasting can allow an individual to get in shape and keep up their weight reduction.

However, not every person should quick. Fasting can be

dangerous for kids, creating adolescents, pregnant ladies, older individuals, and individuals with hidden wellbeing conditions.

10. Counting Calories and Keeping A Nourishment Diary

Counting calories can be a viable method to abstain from gorging. By tallying calories, an individual will know about precisely the amount they are devouring. This mindfulness can assist them with removing superfluous calories and settle on better dietary decisions.

A nourishment diary can enable an individual to consider what and the amount they are devouring each day. By doing this, they can likewise guarantee that they are getting enough of each stimulating nutrition type, for example, vegetables and proteins.

11. Brushing Teeth Between Dinners or Prior at Night

Notwithstanding improving dental cleanliness, brushing the teeth can help lessen the impulse to nibble between dinners.

If an individual who regularly snacks around evening time brushes their teeth prior at night, they may feel less enticed to eat extra snacks.

12. Eating More Fruits and Vegetables

An eating routine wealthy in products of the soil can enable an individual to get more fit and keep up their weight reduction.

The author of an orderly survey supports this case, expressing that advancing an expansion in products of the soil utilization is probably not going to cause any weight increase, even without instructing individuals to diminish their use regarding different nourishments.

13. Lessening Carbohydrate Consumption

Diets low in basic starches can enable an individual to reduce their weight by constraining the measure of added sugar that they eat.

Restorative low carbohydrate abstains from food center around expending entire sugars, high fats, fiber, and lean proteins. Rather than restricting all sugars for a brief period, this ought to be a reasonable, long haul dietary alteration.

14. Eating More Fiber

Fiber offers a few potential advantages to an individual hoping to get thinner. Research in Nutrition expresses that an expansion in fiber utilization can enable an individual to feel fuller more rapidly.

Furthermore, fiber helps weight reduction by advancing absorption and adjusting the microorganisms in the gut.

15. Expanding Traditional Cardiovascular and Resistance Training

Numerous individuals do not practice regularly and may likewise have inactive occupations. It is critical to incorporate both cardiovascular (cardio) work out, for example, running or strolling, and opposition preparing in a regular exercise program.

Cardio enables the body to consume calories rapidly while obstruction preparing manufactures fit bulk. Bulk can assist individuals with consuming more calories very still.

Furthermore, explore has discovered that individuals who take an interest in high-intensity interval training (HIIT) can lose more weight and see more prominent enhancements in their cardiovascular wellbeing than individuals who are utilizing other mainstream strategies for weight reduction.

16. Devouring Whey Protein

Individuals who use whey protein may expand their slender bulk while diminishing muscle versus fat, which can help with weight reduction.

Research from 2014 found that whey protein, in the mix with practice or a weight reduction diet, may help diminish body weight and muscle to fat ratio.

17. Eating Slowly

Eating slowly can enable an individual to decrease all outnumber of calories that they expend in one sitting. The purpose behind this is it can require some investment to understand that the stomach is full.

One examination showed that eating rapidly relates to corpulence. While the investigation couldn't prescribe mediations to enable an individual to eat all the more gradually, the outcomes do propose that eating nourishment at a slower pace can help decrease calorie consumption.

Biting nourishment completely and eating at a table with others may enable an individual to back off while eating.

18.Including Chili

Adding spice to nourishments may enable an individual to get more fit. Capsaicin is a compound that is normally present in flavors, for example, bean stew powder, and may have constructive outcomes.

For instance, inquire about demonstrates that capsaicin can assist ignite with fatting and increment digestion, yet at low rates.

19.Getting More Sleep

There is a link between corpulence and an absence of value rest. The research proposes that getting adequate rest can add to weight loss. The researchers found that ladies who depicted their rest quality as poor or reasonable were more averse to effectively get in shape than the individuals who detailed their rest quality as being generally excellent.

20.   Utilizing a Smaller Plate

Utilizing smaller plates could have a positive mental impact. Individuals will, in general, fill their plate, so lessening the size of the plate may help decrease the measure of nourishment that an individual eats in one sitting. A 2015 systematic reassessment inferred that diminishing plate size could affect partition control and vitality utilization, yet it was hazy whether this was material over the full scope of bit sizes. Individuals hoping to get in shape securely and normally should concentrate on making a perpetual way of life changes instead of embracing brief measures.

Individuals must concentrate on making changes that they can keep up. Now and again, an individual may want to execute changes steadily or take a stab at presenting each in turn.

Any individual who thinks that it is difficult to get more fit may profit by addressing a specialist or dietitian to discover an arrangement that works for them.

Chapter 2: Changing Your Mindset

Why a Rigid and Aggressive Approach Doesn't Work

When it comes to making any sort of change in life, the approach you take will make or break your success. If you choose a strategy that doesn't work well with your specific personality, the likelihood of relapse occurring will be extremely high. We will discuss the drawbacks of approaching change with an aggressive and rigid approach.

Taking an approach that is focused on perfection leaves you feeling down on yourself and like a failure most of the time. Because this causes you to notice that you are not perfect instead of focusing on the right parts, the progress you have made will always make you feel like you are not doing enough or that you have not made enough progress. Since you will never achieve perfection as this is impossible for anyone, you will never feel satisfaction or allow yourself to celebrate your achievements. You must recognize that this will be something complicated, but that you will do it anyways. If you force yourself into change like a drill sergeant and with an aggressive mindset, you will end up beating yourself up every day for something. Pushing yourself will not lead to a long-lasting change, as you will eventually become fed up with all the rules you have placed on yourself, and you will just want to abandon the entire mission. If you approach the change with rigidity, you will not allow yourself time to look back on your achievements and celebrate yourself, to have a tasty meal that is good for your soul every once in a while, and you may fall off of your plan in a more extreme way than you were before. You may end up having a week-long binge and dropping down into worse habits than you had back.

Your mindset plays a huge role in your success when it comes to change. The way that you view your journey will make or break it and will determine whether or not your change is lasting or fleeting, and whether or not you become invested in making the changes in your life. While you need to push yourself to do anything hard, the key is knowing when to ease up on yourself a little bit and when to push harder. Recognizing and responding to this is much more useful than putting your nose to the grindstone every day and becoming burnt out, tired, and left without any more willpower. Continuing on this challenging journey that a lifestyle change involves, you must give yourself a break now and then. Think of this like running a marathon where you will need to go about it slowly and purposefully with a strategy in mind. If you ran into a marathon full-speed and refused to slow down or look back at all, you would lose energy, stamina, and motivation in quite a short amount of time and turn back or run off the side of the road feeling defeated and as if you failed. Looking at this example, you can see that this person did not fail. They just approached the marathon with the wrong strategy and that they would have been completely capable of finishing that marathon if they had taken their time, followed a plan, and slowed down every once in a while, to regain their strength. Even if they walked the marathon slowly for hours and hours, eventually, they would make it over that finish line. They would probably also do so feeling proud, accomplished, and like a new person. This is how we want to view this journey or any journey of self-improvement. Even if you take only one tiny step each day, you are making a step toward your goal, and that is the crucial part.

The Deprivation Trap

There is a term when it comes to dieting that is called The Deprivation Trap. The deprivation trap is something that can occur when you approach dieting with a strict mindset. What this means is that you become stuck in a type of thinking trap within your mind. In this type of thinking, you become focused on what you can't have and what you are restricting yourself off. You become hyper-focused on everything you can't allow yourself to have and become resentful of the fact that you aren't able just to eat what you want. After a while, because you are focusing so intently on what you can't have and the fact that you can't have it, you decide that you are just going to have it anyway, or just have a little bit of it, out of a feeling of anger and entitlement. The next thing you know, you have gone on a binge, and after restricting yourself entirely for some time, you have now undone that in a single sitting. You will then begin to feel terrible about yourself and what you have done, and you begin to feel like you need to punish yourself. Thus can start the cycle of deprivation.

Further, it is quite challenging to avoid this when you are trying to make a change by using deprivation. It is quite rare that a person, no matter how strong their willpower, will be able to deprive themselves of something without easing off of it ultimately. A sudden and strict deprivation is not natural to our brains and will leave us feeling confused and frustrated.

How to Overcome the Deprivation Trap

To avoid the deprivation trap or overcome it if you are already finding yourself there, there are things that we can do and approaches we can take that will set us up better for success.

To avoid this trap, the first thing we must do is prevent complete deprivation of anything. Instead of depriving ourselves of something ultimately, we will instead try to make better choices, one meal or one snack at a time. Focusing on small parts of our day or lower sections of our lives will help us to motivate ourselves. This is because looking forward to the rest of our lives and thinking that we will never be able to have a sure thing again is quite an overwhelming thought, especially if this is something that we enjoy. Therefore, we must instead look at it like "I will make a better choice for my lunch today," and then all you need to focus on is lunch, not the entire rest of your life.

Strategies for the Mind

Like we all know and read in some websites about weight-loss, easing into a lifestyle change is the best way to go about something like this because of the way that our minds work. We don't like looking forward to our lives and feeling like we will have no control over what we are going to do with it. By choosing smaller sections to break it up into, we can be more present in each moment, which makes making healthy choices easier. By doing so, all of these small sections add up to weeks, months, and eventually years of healthy options. Finally, we have gone a year without turning to sweets in a moment of sadness and only chosen them when we are consciously choosing to treat ourselves.

Another strategy that we can use for our minds is to reward yourself at milestones along your journey. At one week you can reward yourself with a date night at a restaurant, or at one month you can visit the new bakery down the street. This not only helps you to stay motivated because you are allowing yourself some of the joys you love, but it also keeps you motivated because you are allowing yourself to take time to look back at how far you have come and feel great about your progress. Allowing yourself to celebrate goes hand in hand with this, as well. When you make the right choice or plan what you will order at a restaurant before you get there, allowing yourself to feel happy and proud is very important. By doing this, you are showing yourself that you have done something great, that you are capable of making changes, and that you will allow yourself to feel good about these positive strides you have made instead of just looking to the next one all the time. If you were to ignore this and be of the mindset that nothing is good enough, you would end up feeling burnt out and entirely down about the length of the process. Think of that marathon analogy again, and this is what can happen if we don't allow ourselves time to feel proud and accomplished for small victories along the way.

Another strategy for the mind is to avoid beating yourself up for falling off the wagon. This may happen sometimes. What we need to do, though, is to focus not on the fact that it has happened, but on how we are going to deal with and react to it. There are a variety of reactions that a person can have to this. We will examine the possible responses and the pros and cons below:

One is that they feel as though their progress is ruined and that they might as well begin another time again, so they go back to their old ways and may not try again for some time. This could happen many times over as they will fall off each time and then decide that they might as well give up this time and try again, but each time it ends the same.

Two, the person could fall off of their diet plan and tell themselves that this day is a write-off and that they will begin the next day again. The problem with this method is that continuing the rest of the day as you would have before you decided to make a change will make it so that the next day is like beginning all over again, and it will be tough to start again. They may be able to start the next day again, and it could be fine, but they must be able to motivate themselves if they are to do this. Knowing that you have fallen off makes it so that you may feel down on yourself and feel as though you can't do it, so beginning again the next day is significant.

And they then decide that they will pick it up again the next week. This will be even harder than starting the next day again as multiple days of eating whatever you like will make it very hard to go back to making the healthy choices still afterwards.

Four, after eating something that they wish they hadn't, and that wasn't a healthy choice, they will decide not to eat anything for the rest of the day so that they don't eat too many calories or too much sugar, and decide that the next day they will begin again. This is very difficult on the body as you are going to be quite hungry by the time bed rolls around. Instead of forgiving yourself, you are punishing yourself, and it will make it very hard not to reach for chips late at night when you are starving and feeling down.

Chapter 3: Why Is It Hard to Lose Weight?

For anyone who has ever struggled with weight, life can seem like an uphill battle. It can be downright devastating to see how difficult it can be to turn things around and shed some weight.

The fact of the matter is that losing weight doesn't have to be an uphill battle. Most of this requires you to understand better why this struggle happens and what you can do to help give yourself a fighting chance.

Physiological factors are affecting your ability to lose weight. There are also psychological, emotional and even spiritual causes that affect your overall body's ability to help you lose weight and reach your ideal weight levels.

The Obvious Culprits

The obvious culprits that are holding you back are diet, a lack of exercise and a combination of both.

First off, your diet plays a crucial role in your overall health and wellbeing. When it comes to weight management, your diet has everything to do with your ability to stay in shape and ward of unwanted weight.

When it comes to diet, we are not talking about keto, vegan, or Atkins; we are talking about the common foods which you consume and the amounts that you have of each one which is why diet is one of the obvious culprits. If you have a diet that is high in fat, high in sodium and high in sugar, you can rest assured that your body will end up gaining weight at a rapid rate.

When you consume high amounts of sugar, carbs and fats, your body transforms them into glucose which storing it in the body as fat. Of course, a proportion of the glucose produced by your body is used up as energy. However, if you consume far more than you need, your body isn't going to get rid of it; your body is going to hold on to it and make sure that it is stored for a rainy day.

Here is another vital aspect to consider: sweet and salty foods, the kind that we love so dearly, trigger "happy hormones" in the brain, namely dopamine. Dopamine is a hormone that is released by the body when it "feels good". And the food is one of the best ways to trigger it, which is why you somehow feel better after eating your favorite meals. It also explains the reason why we resort to food when we are not feeling well, which is called "comfort food", and it is one of the most popular coping mechanisms employed by folks around the world.

This rush of dopamine causes a person to become addicted to food. As with any addiction, there comes a time when you need to get more and more of that same substance to meet your body's requirements.

As a result of diet, a lack of regular exercise can do a number on your ability to lose weight and maintain a healthy balance. What regular exercise does is increase your body's overall caloric requirement. As such, your metabolism needs to convert fat at higher rates to keep up with your body's energy demands.

As the body's energetic requirements increase, that is, as your exercise regimen gets more and more intense, you will find that you will need increased amounts of both oxygen and glucose which is one of the reasons why you feel hungrier when you ramp up your workouts.

However, increased caloric intake isn't just about consuming more and more calories for the sake of consuming more and more calories; you need to consume an equal amount of proteins, carbs, fats and vitamins too for your body to build the necessary elements that will build muscle, foster movement and provide proper oxygenation in the blood.

Moreover, nutrients are required for the body to recover. One of the byproducts of exercise is called "lactic acid". Lactic acid builds up in the muscles as they get more and more tired. Lactic acid signals the body that it is time to stop working out or risk injury if you continue. Without lactic acid, your body would have no way of knowing when your muscles have overextended their capacity.

After you have completed your workout, the body needs to get rid of the lactic acid buildup. So, if you don't have enough of the right minerals in your body, for example, potassium, your muscles will ache for days until your body is finally able to get rid of the lactic acid buildup. This example goes to show how proper nutrition is needed to help the body get moving and also recover once it is done exercising.

As a result, a lack of exercise reconfigures your body's metabolism to work at a slower pace. What that means is that you need to consume fewer calories to fuel your body's lack of exercise. So, if you end up wasting more than you need, your body will just put it away for a rainy day. Plain and simple.

The Sneaky Culprits

The sneaky culprits are the ones that aren't quite so overt in causing you to gain weight or have trouble shedding pounds. These culprits hide beneath the surface but are very useful when it comes to keeping you overweight. The first culprit we are going to be looking at is called "stress".

Stress is a potent force. From an evolutionary perspective, it exists as a means of fueling the flight-or-fight response. Stress is the human response to danger. When a person senses danger, the body begins to secrete a hormone called "cortisol". When cortisol begins running through the body, it signals the entire system to prep for a potential showdown. Depending on the situation, it might be best to hightail it out and live to fight another day.

In our modern way of life, stress isn't so much a response to life and death situations (though it can certainly be). Instead, it is the response to cases that are deemed as "conflictive" by the mind. This could be a confrontation with a co-worker, bumper to bumper traffic, or any other type of situation in which a person feels vulnerable in some way.

Throughout our lives, we subject to countless interactions in which we must deal with stress. In general terms, the feelings of alertness subside when the perceived threat is gone. However, when a person is exposed to prolonged periods of stress, any number of changes can happen.

One such change is overexposure to cortisol. When there is too much cortisol in the body, the body's overall response is to hoard calories, increase the production of other hormones such as adrenaline and kick up the immune system's function.

This response by the body is akin to the panic response that the body would assume when faced with prolonged periods of hunger or fasting. As a result, the body needs to go into survival mode. Please bear in mind that the body has no clue if it is being chased by a bear, dealing with a natural disaster or just having a bad day at the office. Regardless of the circumstances, the body is faced with the need to ensure its survival. So, anything that it eats goes straight to fat stores.

Moreover, a person's stressful situation makes them search for comfort and solace. There are various means of achieving this. Food is one of them. So is alcohol consumption. These two types of pleasures lead to significant use of calories. Again, when the body is in high gear, it will store as many calories and keep them in reserve.

This what makes you gain weight when you are stressed out.

Another of the sneaky culprits is sleep deprivation. In short, sleep deprivation is sleeping less than the recommended 8 hours that all adults should sleep. In the case of children, the recommended amount of sleep can be anywhere from 8 to 12 hours, depending on their age.

Granted, some adults can function perfectly well with less than 8 hours' sleep. Some folks can work perfectly well with

6 hours' sleep while there are folks who are shattered when they don't get eight or even more hours' sleep. This is different for everyone as each individual is different in this regard.

That being said, sleep deprivation can trigger massive amounts of cortisol. This, fueled by ongoing exposure to stress, leads the body to further deepening its panic mode. When this occurs, you can rest assured that striking a healthy balance between emotional wellbeing and physical health can be nearly impossible to achieve.

Now, the best way to overcome sleep deprivation is to get sleep. But that is easier said than done. One of the best ways to get back on track to a certain degree is to get in enough sleep when you can.

The last sneaky culprit on our list is emotional distress. Emotional distress can occur as a result of any number of factors. For example, the loss of a loved one, a stressful move, a divorce, or the loss of a job can all contribute to large amounts of emotional distress. While all the situations mentioned above begin as a stressful situation, they can fester and lead to severe psychological issues. Over time, these emotional issues can grow into more profound topics such as General Anxiety Disorder or Depression. Studies have shown that prolonged periods of stress can lead to depression and a condition known as Major Depression.

The most common course of treatment for anxiety and depression is the use of an antidepressant. And guess what: one of the side effects associated with antidepressants is the weight. The reason for this is that antidepressant tinkers with the brain's chemistry in such a way that they alter the brain's processing of chemicals through the suppression of serotonin transport. This causes the brain to readjust its overall chemistry. Thus, you might find the body unable to process food quite the same way. In general, it is common to see folks gain as much as 10 pounds as a result of taking antidepressants.

As you can see, weight gain is not the result of "laziness" or being "undisciplined". Sure, you might have to clean up your diet somewhat and get more exercise. But the causes we have outlined here ought to provide you with enough material to see why there are less obvious causes that are keeping yours from achieving your ideal weight. This is why meditation plays such a key role in helping you deal with stress and emotional strife while helping you find a balance between your overall mental and physical wellbeing.

Ultimately, the strategies and techniques that we will further outline here will provide you with the tools that will help you strike that balance and eventually lead you to find the most effective way in which you will deal with the rigors of your day-to-day life while being able to make the most out of your efforts to lead a healthier life. You have everything you need to do it. So, let's find out how you can achieve this.

Chapter 4: Why You Should Stop Emotional Eating

We don't know we're an emotional eater for most of us, or we don't think it's that severe. For some of us, it doesn't lead to feelings of shame or weight gain. We can console some of us and think it's not a big deal, but it's not.

Among others, emotional eating is out of balance, something that can dominate our everyday lives. This may seem like overwhelming cravings or hunger, but it's just the feeling that we feel hungry, helpless and add to our weight.

Comfort food gives us immediate pleasure and takes away feeling. Digestion and sensation require a lot of time, and the body can't do it. Comfort eating helps us to suppress pain because we flood our digestive tract with poisonous waste.

When we feel anxious, feeling a big empty hole inside us like we're hungry can be natural. Instead of confronting what this means—i.e. our emotions—we're stuffing it down. In culture, it seems we are afraid to feel too much that we don't even know we're running from our feelings much of the time.

If we don't let ourselves react, we'll repress it. You will feel exhausted until you begin to let yourself feel the thoughts or feelings that emerge and avoid stuffing down. It is because the body releases past pent-up emotions, and it can strike you hard.

That's why it can be hard to let go of emotional eating, as we have to conquer the initial "scare" to move on and start learning to accept emotions for what they are. To be present, allowing a feeling to wash over us is wonderful and should be appreciated.

The more you allow yourself to be in the present moment and feel, the fewer feelings that overtake you, the less terrified you will be. The emotion's strength also decreases. You'll become mentally and physically stronger. When it's off your stomach, you'll feel so much better than replacing it with food.

Getting to this point isn't fast. Some people can split their emotional eating by better nourishing their bodies to get rid of physical cravings and supporting others when they feel anxious or emotional.

To stop emotional eating, you must be mindful of how and why you eat—taking a day out to consider what makes you happy. Many people don't even understand real hunger! When you're eating mentally, can you stop yourself?

Could you sit and let the emotion wash over you instead of

eating, give yourself time to feel it and transfer it? Or would you talk to someone about how you feel?

Don't injure yourself.

Emotional eating is usually something you've done from an early age because it's part of your make-up. It's a practiced habit, so you've learned to cope with the environment.

It takes time to undo something so ingrained in you, so if you find yourself eating out of guilt, if you mess up, learn from it, just move on. Recognition is the first step. If you know you eat safely, you can conquer it.

Journaling will also help you recognize eating habits. Note down before, during and after a meal. What caused eating was real hunger?

To learn how to avoid emotional eating, I can help. For years, I suffered from an emotional eating epidemic, sometimes going on a day-to-day binge eating marathon. I never really understood what caused these eating outbursts, all I knew was that I would start eating and not stop until the food was gone, or anyone near me saw me.

The situation escalated, and my weight started to increase. Any diet I was on would instantly fail, and my self-confidence reached an all-time low. My eating causes were thought to be related to work stress, but so many others may play a part. Relationships, depression, financial difficulties, and many others will easily consume binge sequence.

When I started trying to figure out how to avoid emotional eating, I didn't know where to start. Like you, I went online and started investigating. I spent the whole day reading, digesting, and gathering emotional cure knowledge, then around 3 a.m. I found my savior that morning.

And how can you avoid emotional eating?

The answer is very easy. The trick is identifying the real root cause of the problems and addressing those root causes. You may think its tension or job issues. Yet mental eating disorders are also much more profound than on the surface. Following the root, a cause can quickly treat these symptoms and safely cure your binge eating.

Mental eating satisfies your mental appetite. It's not about your kitchen, but the issue lies in your head. What are the most powerful emotional eating challenge strategies?

List your food cravings to relax.

Distracting yourself doesn't mean being lazy in this situation. It's not like texting while driving, or you're out of control. When you hide from your food cravings, it means you're turning your focus to something else. It's more purposeful.

Do something or concentrate on another action or event. Whenever you feel like gorging food, try getting a piece of paper and list five items from five categories of something like the names of five people whenever you feel upset, angry or depressed.

Perhaps you should mention five ways to relax. If you want to calm down, what are your five places?

When anxious, what five feel-good phrases can you tell yourself? How about five things to stop eating?

Place on your fridge or kitchen cabinet after finishing this list. Next time you're overwhelmed by your persuasive food cravings, browse through your list and do one of the 25 things suggested there.

Prepare ahead for future emotional issues.

Over the weekend, grab a piece of paper and a pencil and take a path to your tasks in the days ahead. Your map reveals your expected exits and potential detours. Pick an emotionally consuming picture.

Place the icon over an event or activity that could cause your food cravings, like an early lunch with your in-laws. Prepare ahead for that case. Search for the restaurant menu online to order something delicious and nutritious.

Drop the concerns inside.

Whenever anxious, taking a deep breath helps. Another thing to detoxify yourself from stress is to do a visual trick. Breathe deeply and imagine a squeegee (that piece of cloth you use to clean your window or windshield) near your eyes. Slowly breathe out, picture the squeegee wiping clean inside. Delete all your concerns. Do it three times.

Self-talk like you're royalty. Self-criticism is usually emotional. Toxic words you say to yourself, such as "I'm such a loser" or "I can never seem to do anything right," force you to drive to the nearest. Don't be fooled by these claims, though brief.

Such feelings, like acid rain, slowly erode your well-being. The next time you're caught telling yourself these negative things, overcome by moving to a third-person perspective.

If you think "I'm such a mess," tell yourself then that "Janice is such a mess, but Janice will do what it takes to get things done and make herself happy."

This approach will get you out of the negative self-talk loop and have some perspective. Pull up and be positive and have the strength and avoid emotional eating.

Over-food is still not given enough consideration. It's always seen as not a serious problem to laugh at.

This is an incorrect view as a horrific condition needing urgent treatment. The positive thing is that you take action to help you avoid emotional eating forever. I know because I did it myself.

Step1-Recognize triggers

For each person, emotional eating is triggered differently. Some people get cravings when stressed out, some when depressed or bored. You need to try to work out the emotional causes. When you know what they are, you'll get an early notice when the urge to feed comes to you.

Step 2-Eliminate Temptation

One thing most people don't realize about emotional eating is that desire is always for one specific food. It's always ice-cream or candy for kids. It's still pizza for guys.

When you couldn't fulfil this lure, it won't bother you. Save your home from all of these temptations.

Throw out any nearby pizza delivery locations. Again, you know your tempters, so get rid of them and make overeating difficult.

Step 3-Break contact

It's instant and urgent when craving hits. You're fed RIGHT NOW! To stop this, you must break this immediate bond by taking some time between desires and eating.

Call a friend Count to 60

Write down what you feel like

Do some exercises go out for a walk

Take a shower

What you can do to make the urge subside do wonder.

Take these three moves, and you'll soon take them better and conquer emotional eating for good.

Chapter 5: Hypnotic Gastric Band Techniques

If you would like to lose some weight without using surgery, then the hypnotic gastric band is the best tool for you. The hypnotic gastric band is the natural healthy eating tool that will help to control your appetite and your portion sizes. In this sense, hypnosis plays a significant role in helping you to lose weight without having to go through the risk that comes with surgery.

It is a subconscious suggestion that you already have, a gastric band comes intending to influence the body to respond by creating a feeling of satiety. It is now available in a public domain that dieting does not help to solve lifestyle challenges that are needed for weight loss and management.

Temporary diet plans are not effective while maintaining continuous plans are difficult. Notably, these plans are going to deprive you of your favorite foods, since they are too restrictive. Deep down within you, you might have a problem with your body's weight since diets have not worked for you in the past.

If you want to try something that will be able to provide a

positive edge for you, then you should be able to control your cravings around food hypnotically. By reaching this point, you must try hypnosis, which has proven some results in aiding weight loss.

So now you can relax and take this time to wind yourself down and allow all those tensions to start flowing out and disappearing. So just bring to mind to remember that hypnosis is just self-hypnosis, that this is not something that someone will be able to do for you. Because hypnosis is simply a state of deep relaxation, which successfully helps you to bypass your critical factors so that the suggestions that are beneficial to your true self will be readily received and accepted by your deeper unconscious mind.

After all, trance is an everyday natural calming experience, and you are entering into that experience easily and effortlessly. So start by asking yourself, if you've ever put yourself in a calm relaxing state before this moment, and if so, you can recall all those calm and relaxing states that you've previously experienced, whether it's via your favorite hobby, an activity, a journey or a holiday.

The most important thing to realize is that you should bring to your mind, relaxation, and protective magical thinking practices each day in your waking state because you know that the practice imprints it in your mind. And as time goes by, it becomes easier for you to be able to gain the benefits of these experiences, which helps to promote self-acceptance.

Once they become permanently fixed into your mind, you will experience some positive changes in your life, and they will become active by helping you to create positive changes in your life that are for your benefit, and they will lead you forward towards a real realization of those changes. And as you speak directly to the deeper inner part of the self that controls, you're eating habits and weight, you will realize that you have been eating more food than the food that your body wants or needs. And you will realize that your mind controls you're eating habits.

Now just seeing all those levers that you can adjust; you can then choose which one to use because you know that you have the power over your weight and you're eating habits. And also, you know what you're eating. The exact time and amount that you choose to eat are controlled in this place, which is the deeper part of your authentic self.

This part of the body is not your stomach or your appetite, but it controls your food, but it is your mind, and you get to ask that aspect of yourself beginning today, to develop new habits for yourself. And set new positive goals for yourself because you are laying a mental foundation for yourself, who is now a cheerful, attractive, positive, and authentic you. The great importance of this new you and your healthy, active, and attractive body is that you are eating less food, and you are happier.

The more you smile, and the more relaxed you are, the better you will look and the better you will feel. Also, you will be able to find satisfaction in eating less and pride yourself in knowing that each time you do so, you are rewarding your slimmer, healthier, and natural self. And you will know that the slimmer you are deep within you as you exercise, this new strength will grow. And as you eat healthily and sensibly, you will find yourself filling satisfied, and you will discover that the exercise makes it more reinforce and more natural towards your authentic identity.

Because it is like using and strengthening your muscles to become stronger and stronger, now eating sensibly becomes easier, easier, in a practical, and the positive way means that you are mentally asking your body the foods it needs, and then you are taking the time to listen to your own body quietly. And always check in with your body on the little food that your body needs from time to time, and you will be able to take time to integrate these ideas on a deeper level.

If you are listening to these and choosing to drift into a deeper sleep, you can just do so. Now just feeling good will allow your body to be able to drift down and go into a deeper and restful sleep. If you want to get up and continue with your activities, then you have to count from one to five, and when you reach five, you can then open your eyes and come back to the fully conscious reality.

And so, on counting one, you should allow yourself to come back to full conscious reality with relaxation and ease. Then as you count two, come back slowly to your full conscious reality, and as you count three, take some nice deep relaxing breath. Moreover, as you count four, allow your eyes to open as if you've bathed them with fresh water, and now, as you count five, open your eyes completely and adjust yourself to your environment while getting ready to carry on with your day's activity.

Remember to use words that resonate with you. The affirmations need not be empty for you. They ought to have a close relation and meaning attached to them. The proper statements for the appropriate situation goes a long way in achieving success.

You can try repeating your affirmations before you go to bed. As the brain gets ready to go on "autopilot" mode, the subconscious mind becomes more active, thereby absorbing the last bits of information for the day. Repeating affirmations before you sleep not only makes you slip into dreamland in a more confident and relaxed state but also helps to convince the mind.

You might begin to wonder why, if affirmations work, they are not used to get out of "tricky" situations. For example, if you are feeling sick, would you proceed to state, "I am cured. I am well,"? Affirmations work best with an aligned state of mind. If you believe to be well, it is more likely that you will notice a decline in symptoms. If you do not believe in your affirmations, you will continue to battle through the temperature and other physical discomforts.

Finding the right words to use can be a stroll in the park; however, remembering to repeat these words, severally could present itself as a challenge. The other obstacle you might face is having two conflicting thoughts. One of them is the carefully considered affirmation, while the other is a counterproductive negation. Try the best you can to disprove the negative thoughts but do not feed them time nor energy. It will be quite challenging to believe affirmations too at the beginning. However, as time goes on, it will become easier to convince yourself. Practice makes perfect.

Chapter 6: Preparing Your Body for Your Hypnotic Gastric Band

The physical gastric band requires a surgical procedure that involves reducing the size of your stomach pocket to accommodate a less volume of food and as a result of the stretching of the walls of the stomach, send signals to the brain that you are filled and therefore need to stop eating any further.

The hypnotic gastric band also works in the same manner, although in this case the only surgical tools you will need are your mind and your body and the great part is, you can conduct the procedure yourself. The hypnotic gastric band also conditions your mind and body to restrict excess consumption of food after very modest meals. There are three specific differences between the surgical (physical), and hypnotic gastric bands:

- In using the hypnotic band, all necessary adjustments are done by continued use of trance.
- There is an absence of physical surgery and

therefore you are exposed to no risks at all.

- When compared with the surgical gastric band, the hypnotic gastric band is a lot cheaper and easier to do.

How Hypnosis Improves Communication Between Stomach and Brain

How would you know when you have had enough to eat? Initially, you will begin to feel the weight and area of the food. When your stomach is full, the food presses against and extends the stomach well, and the nerve endings in the walls of the stomach respond. When these nerves are stimulated, they transfer a signal to the brain, and we get the feeling of satiety.

Sadly, when individuals always overeat, they become desensitized to both the nerve signals and the neuropeptide signaling system. During the initial installation trance, we use hypnotic and images to re-sensitize the brain to these signs. Your hypnotic band restores the full effect of these nervous and neuropeptide messages. With the benefits of hypnotic in view, we can recalibrate this system and increase your sensitivity to these signs, so you feel full and truly satisfied when you have eaten enough to fill that little pouch at the top of your stomach.

A hypnotic gastric band causes your body to carry on precisely as if you have carried out a surgical operation. It contracts your stomach and adjusts the signals from your stomach to your brain, so you feel full rapidly. The hypnotic band uses a few uncommon attributes of hypnotic. As a matter of first importance, hypnotic permits us to talk to parts of the body and mind that are not under conscious control. Interestingly, as it might appear, in a trance, we can really convince the body to carry on distinctively even though our conscious mind has no methods for coordinating that change.

The Power of The Gastric Band

A renowned and dramatic case of the power of hypnotic to influence our bodies directly is in the emergency treatment of burns. A few doctors have used hypnotic on many occasions to accelerate and improve the recuperating of extreme injuries and to help reduce the excruciating pains for his patients. If somebody is seriously burnt, there will be damage to the tissue, and the body reacts with inflammation. The patients are hypnotized to forestall the soreness. His patients heal quite rapidly and with less scarring.

There are a lot more instances of how the mind can directly and physically influence the body. We realize that chronic stress can cause stomach ulcers, and a psychological shock can turn somebody's hair to grey color overnight. In any case, what I especially like about this aspect of hypnotism is that it is an archived case of how the mind influences the body positively and medically. It will be somewhat of a miraculous event if the body can get into a hypnotic state that can cause significant physical changes in your body. Hypnotic trance without anyone else has a profound physiological effect. The most immediate effect is that subjects discover it deeply relaxing. Interestingly, the most widely recognized perception that my customers report after I have seen them— regardless of what we have been dealing with—is that their loved ones tell them they look more youthful.

Cybernetic Loop

Your brain and body are in constant correspondence in a cybernetic loop: they continually influence one another. As the mind unwinds in a trance, so too does the body. When the body unwinds, it feels good, and it sends that message to the brain, which thus feels healthier and unwinds much more. This procedure decreases stress and makes more energy accessible to the immune system of the body. It is essential to take note that the remedial effects of hypnotic don't require tricks or amnesia. For example, burns patients realize they have been burnt, so they don't need to deny the glaring evidence of how burnt parts of their bodies are. He essentially hypnotizes them and requests that they envision cool, comfortable sensations over the burnt area. That imaginative activity changes their body's response to the burns.

The enzymes that cause inflammation are not released, and accordingly, the burn doesn't advance to a more elevated level of damage, and there is reduced pain during the healing process.

By using hypnotic and imagery, a doctor can get his patients' bodies to do things that are totally outside their conscious control. Willpower won't make these sorts of changes, but the creative mind is more grounded than the will. By using hypnotic and imagery to talk to the conscious mind, we can have a physiological effect in as little as 20 minutes. In my work, I recently had another phenomenal idea of how hypnotic can accelerate the body's normal healing process. I worked with a soldier in the special forces who experienced extreme episodes of skin inflammation (eczema). He revealed to me that the quickest recuperation he had ever made from an eczema episode was six days. I realized that the way toward healing is a natural sequence of events carried out by various systems within the body, so I hypnotized him and, while in a trance requested that his conscious mind follow precisely the same process that it regularly uses to heal his eczema, however, to do everything quicker.

One and a half days after, the eczema was gone. With hypnotic, we can enormously enhance the effect of the mind. When we fit your hypnotic gastric band, we are using the very same strategy of hypnotic correspondence to the conscious mind. We communicate to the brain with distinctive imagery, and the brain alters your body's responses, changing your physical response to food so your stomach is constricted, and you feel truly full after only a few.

What Makes the Hypnotic Work So Well?

A few people think that it is difficult to accept that trance and imagery can have such an extreme and ground-breaking effect. Some doctors were at first distrustful and accepted that his patients more likely than not had fewer burns than was written in their medical records, because the cures he effected had all the earmarks of being close to marvelous. It took quite a long while, and numerous exceptional remedies before such work were generally understood and acknowledged.

Occasionally, the cynic and the patient are the same individuals. We need the results, but we battle to accept that it truly will work. At the conscious level, our minds are very much aware of the contrast between what we imagine and physical reality. In any case, another astounding hypnotic marvel shows that it does not make a difference what we accept at the conscious level since trance permits our mind to react to a reality that is independent of what we deliberately think. This phenomenon is classified as "trance logic."

Trance logic was first recognized 50 years ago by a renowned researcher of hypnotic named Dr. Martin Orne, who worked for a long time at the University of Pennsylvania. Dr. Orne directed various tests that demonstrated that in hypnotic, individuals could carry on as though two absolutely opposing facts were valid simultaneously. In one study, he hypnotized a few people so they couldn't see a seat he put directly before them. Then he requested that they walk straight ahead. The subjects all swerved around the seat.

Notwithstanding, when examined regarding the chair, they reported there was nothing there. They couldn't see the seat. Some of them even denied that they had served by any means. They accepted they were telling the truth when they said they couldn't see the seat, but at another level, their bodies realized it was there and moved to abstain from hitting it.

The test showed that hypnotic permits the mind to work at the same time on two separate levels, accepting two isolated, opposing things. It is possible to be hypnotized and have a hypnotic gastric band fitted but then to "know" with your conscious mind that you don't have surgical scars, and you don't have a physical gastric band embedded. Trance logic implies that a part of your mind can trust one thing, and another part can accept the direct opposite, and your mind and body can continue working, accepting that two unique things are valid. So, you will be capable to consciously realize that you have not paid a huge amount of dollars for a surgical process, but then at the deepest level of unconscious command, your body accepts that you have a gastric band and will act in like manner. Subsequently, your stomach is conditioned to signal "feeling full" to your brain after only a couple of mouthfuls. So, you feel satisfied, and you get to lose more weight.

Visualization Is Easier Than You Think

The hypnotic we use to make your gastric band uses "visualization" and "influence loaded imager." Visualization is the creation of pictures in your mind. We would all be able to do it. It is an interesting part of the reasoning. For instance, think about your front door and ask yourself which side the lock is on. To address that question, you see an image in your mind's eye. It doesn't make a difference at all how reasonable or bright the image is, it is only how your mind works, and you see as much as you have to see. Influence loaded imagery is the psychological term for genuinely significant pictures. In this process, we use pictures in the mind's eye that have emotional significance.

Although hypnotic recommendations are incredible, they are dramatically upgraded by ground-breaking images when we are communicating directly to the body. For instance, you will be unable to accelerate your heart just by telling it to beat faster. Still, if you envision remaining on a railroad line and seeing a train surging towards you, your heart accelerates pretty quickly. Your body overreacts to clear, meaningful pictures.

It doesn't make a difference whether you are listening intentionally, your conscious mind will hear all it needs to recreate the real band, in a similar way that a clear image of a moving toward train rushing towards your influences your pulse rate. You do not have to hold the pictures of the operational procedures in your conscious mind, because during an activity you are anesthetized and unconscious. Notwithstanding what you intentionally recollect, underneath the hypnotic anesthesia, your conscious mind uses this information and imagery to introduce your gastric band in the right spot.

Chapter 7: How Negative Emotions Affect Weight Loss

It appears everybody nowadays is attempting to lose weight. We are modified by our condition to look, dress, and even act in a specific way.

Each time you get a magazine, turn on the TV or check out yourself, you are reminded of it. You start to hate your body losing control, disappointed, focused on, apprehensive, and now and again even discouraged.

If losing weight is tied in with eating fewer calories than your body needs and doing some activity to support your digestion, at that point why are such a significant number of individuals as yet attempting to lose weight?

Losing weight has to do with your considerations and convictions as much as it has to do with what you eat. Give me a chance to give you a model. You are staring at the TV, and an advertisement is shown demonstrating a chocolate cheddar cake that you can make utilizing just 3 fixings. You weren't hungry previously, however, since you have seen that cheddar cake you might feel denied and you need to eat. Your feelings are revealing to you that you have to eat, although your stomach isn't disclosing to you that you are hungry.

This is called passionate eating. It is our feelings that trigger our practices.

You may find that when you are feeling focused or depressed, you have this need to eat something since it solaces you somehow or another. The issue is that generally; it isn't healthy that you get for and once you have done this a couple of times it turns into a passionate stay; so every time that you experience pressure or grief, it triggers you to eat something.

Grapples keep you attached to convictions that you have about your life and yourself that prevent you from pushing ahead. You regularly compensate yourself with things that prevent you from losing weight. When you're utilizing nourishment to reward or repay yourself, you are managing stays.

Although the grapples that I am alluding to around passionate eating are not healthy ones, they can likewise be utilized intentionally to get a specific outcome.

Enthusiastic eating doesn't happen because you are physically hungry. It occurs because something triggers a craving for nourishment. You are either intuitively or deliberately covering a hidden, enthusiastic need.

The fear of eating can assume control over your life. It

expends your musings; depleting you of your vitality and self-discipline, making you separate and gorge. This will create more fear and make matters more regrettable.

So how might you conquer your fear and different feelings around eating?

You can transform the majority of your feelings around eating into another more beneficial relationship.

In all actuality, you have a soul. You should find it. It is that spot inside of you that is continually cherishing, forgiving and tranquil. It's a spot that speaks to your higher self.... the genuine you.... the sheltered, loved and entire you. When you find this, the resentment, dissatisfaction, and stress that you are feeling about your weight will vanish.

Things never appear to happen as fast as we might want them to... perhaps your body isn't changing as quickly as you need. This may demoralize you, giving you further reason to indulge.

Comprehend that your body is a gift, and afterward, you will begin to contemplate it.

Quit harping on your stomach fat, your fat arms and butt, your enormous thighs that you hate and every one of the calories that you're taking in, and see all that your body is, all that your body can do and all that your body is doing... right now.

This new mindfulness will make love and acknowledgment for your body such that you never had. You start to treasure it like the astounding gift that it is and center around giving it wellbeing every day in each moment, with each breath.

Begin concentrating on picking up wellbeing as opposed to losing weight, and you will be progressively happy, alive, and thankful. Find the delight of carrying on with a healthy life and feeding your soul consistently. Develop increasingly more love with your body and yourself, and this love will move and transform you from the inside out.

When you tap into an option that is greater than you, you have the constant motivation, which is far more dominant than any battle of the mind or feelings. Tolerating and adoring your body precisely as it is correct presently is the thing that sends the mending vibrations that will quiet your mind and transform your body from the inside out.

When you figure out how to love and acknowledge your body, you are in arrangement with your higher self, that adoring and inviting self.

Grasp what your identity is and not who you think you are or ought to be. Understand the endeavors that you make are seeds. Try not to see the majority of your efforts to lose weight as disappointments, consider them to be seeds you are planting towards progress.

Pardon yourself. Try not to thrash yourself, regardless of how frequently you think you've fizzled, irrespective of what you resemble at this moment and irrespective of how often you need that new beginning. Pardon yourself!

Emotional Weight Loss

Most overeating is emotional!

Not many people understand that they are eating for emotional reasons, and after that, follow specific problems behind their eating to attempt to cure them. If you are an overeater, you have to comprehend the reasons why you overeat, which will enable you to change your eating habits. If not, you wind up stalling out in a foolish cycle like this one; "You overeat because you're disturbed, you put on weight because you overeat, you get steamed because you've put on weight." And you never appear to break out the cycle long enough to lose weight or keep weight off.

If you have numerous pounds to lose, you must understand that your life can be such a considerable amount of superior to anything it is right at this point. If you're not content with yourself, you sure don't need to acknowledge yourself the way you are. Nobody's ideal, and we, as a whole, have problems. Everybody has something to improve in their lives, whether it's changing a harmful habit or getting more fit; the best way to accomplish is beating negative speculation by a positive attitude.

Time and again, we will, in general, discover valid justifications to justify ourselves.

For unknown reasons, many people won't concede the genuine cause of their overeating and will come up with a wide range of reasons, for example, "My parents are fat, so that's why I'm fat, it's innate." or "I have a difficult metabolism, it's so moderate." Making excuses not to eat right or exercise consistently is just a way to justifying why you can't change.

Do We Acquire Fat?

You grow up not realizing the right way to eat, and you grow up overweight. It's a decent wager that your overeating habits are indistinguishable from your folks' and that your figure much takes after theirs. What truly happens is that we acquire the terrible eating habits of those we grow up with. While obesity is once in a while genetic, it tends to be controlled by great eating habits, exercise, and a positive mental attitude.

What Is Metabolism, And How Can It Influence Your Body?

You eat food, the body at that point experiences a procedure of separating all the food and transforming it into usable energy to prop you up. To keep up a healthy weight, you have to adjust your energy IN and your energy OUT. More "in" than "out" = overweight problems. Most of us have a regularly controlled metabolism, yet many need to believe it's delayed as a reason for their weight gain. For an excessive number of people, the aftereffect of inactive living is a losing fight against those extra pounds. Through moderate day by day exercise, you will eat less and, in this manner, lose the extra pounds.

Others may state, "I can't bear to be slim."

Our general stores are loaded up with advantageous, dull plastic foods. Shopping baskets are flooded with precooked, instant, solidified foods with lost dietary benefits. These are high-cost and high-fattening foods. You can bear to eat right, and you can't manage the cost of not to!

Emotional eaters will utilize food to deal with their feelings because of food assuages pressure. When concentrating on food, it occupies our psyches from awkward feelings (fatigue, stress, tension, loneliness) that we would preferably not endure. We go after food whenever we don't like ourselves, and emotional eating turns into an imbued habit.

The initial step is to make sense of what triggers your emotional eating and figure out how to manage the stresses and stress that cause your overeating. Make sense of why you are baffled or upset and start searching for a cure to the problem. Whatever is annoying you rationally need some natural air, not a pack of chips. Work them out. Examine them with family or companions, and if you would prefer not to discuss it, accomplish something, get dynamic.

Start understanding yourself and your needs. Before going after another bit of cake, ask yourself, "Am I extremely eager?" or before you naturally pop something into your mouth, continue asking yourself, "Why am I feeling hungry?" Learn to perceive your appetite. Try not to be terrified to address yourself and get to the base of the problem.

Keep a food diary. By following you're eating habits, it will enable you to see your utilization level and comprehend what triggers your binges. Cause a rundown of different things you can do. Have a go at taking a walk, cleaning the house, working out, calling a companion or tune in to music.

Never center around dieting or weight misfortune!

If you feel wild around food, quit being fixated on your

weight. Most diets expect you to boycott your preferred foods, leaving you unsatisfied and setting off negative feelings. Diet hardship sets up desires and causes you to eat more than you truly need to. Disregard dieting and spotlight on self-care, eating admirably, and being fit.

Begin concentrating on changing your lifestyle habits by eating well, practicing consistently while keeping a positive attitude. The day you quit being fixated on your weight will be the day of your prosperity. Keep in mind a specific something, you have control over your life, and it's your choice to change your lifestyle. You're justified, despite all the trouble!

Chapter 8: Weight Control Individualization

Individualization of a particular program is being stressed, and more of this is still going to happen. If you want the plan you choose to work with to be most effective and produce beautiful results, you must make it yours and ensure that it is unique to you according to what you think can work well for you. Do not start using a program that is not individualized, one that you pick from anywhere and start using because it may not work for you. As you already know, as an individual, you have a unique retinal pattern, fingerprints, and the body chemistry you have does not match that of anyone else. The things you have experienced in life are also different from those of other people.

In the same way, a program that you can use to help you in attaining a unique bodyweight should also be unique to you so that it can achieve maximum positive results. This is why you can see that here you are only provided with a few meditation exercises that you have the chance to choose the best ones that suits you. Giving you so many meditation exercises may be overwhelming when it comes to choosing the activity that suits your body and the one that you are comfortable with. When you are overwhelmed with many choices of meditation exercises to choose from, there is the possibility that you may be confused about making the right decision. Also, you can see that no meditation has been given in a stone manner, the only part that you need to put a lot of effort to ensure success is maintaining your discipline and telling yourself that you know the kind of goals you want. It would be best if you achieved them no matter what happens as you proceed with these exercises.

As an individual, you should discover which form suits you best and follow that diligently until you get the results that you aim for. Many people all over the world have tried meditation methods. Still, many of them have failed because most teachers for meditational schools believe that there is one way to meditate, which applies to each and everyone throughout the world. Many think that they have learned this method from their meditation schools and their teacher through coincidence and by being curious. But the truth is that this could be their best meditation method as individuals, but it does not mean everyone else will find it comfortable, and by using it, they must achieve success. Such kinds of people who have been disappointed because they did not get the results they expected from the meditation exercises belief that it cannot work for them, yet they have not tried other forms of meditation and see how it can work for them.

However, particular aspects come in all forms of meditational paths. For example, meditators should try to continually arrive at the maximum attention possible, which is called coherent attention in some meditational schools. This is whereby, as an individual, you decide to discipline your mind and ensure always to do one thing at a particular time to maintain focus and avoid being overwhelmed. You also decide that you love yourself, and you will treat yourself in a manner that you have promised yourself. These are some of the constants when it comes to various meditational schools. Apart from these, the other things that are involved like doing your meditation while walking in the area of your comfort, do it while sitting in an armchair, and lying on the floor are things that you should decide for yourself and consider the one that you are comfortable with. When it comes to deciding the best time for you to perform the meditational exercises; it is up to you, and there is no conventional way in which you should follow. You can choose to be doing it either once or twice in a day and perform them for one, two, or three weeks depending on what you have promised yourself that you will achieve.

As you continue, if you find that you are committed, and you have a great desire to achieve the healthy body weight that you need to have, you can decide to follow all the meditational exercises because overall, they will help you to achieve your goals. If you do not want to try different meditational paths, then you can decide to go for the combined meditations that you have explicitly identified. There are various forms of meditations that you can choose to go with. Some of these meditational paths include those that stress on the intellectual path, that those enable you to work through emotions and others that have been devised by religious groups in the western world. It does not matter the form of meditation that you have decided to use to attain your goals and experience fulfilment. The truth is that to achieve what you want with these various kinds of meditations. You must put in the work that is required. The results will not be easy for any form of meditation that you decide to go with. Be sure that whatever path you choose, you will not find any easy path because achieving the growth and development you want is difficult. The only best way to achieve what you want is that you be serious and be prepared to put an effort that will not stop soon.

These statements may seem to be put strongly, but those who have attempted to change their lives and succeeded can attest to this and tell you that it is the truth. When we work to achieve a healthy body weight through meditation, we need to know that we will not only individualize our meditational programs but also there are other aspects of our lives that we should also individualize. We will look at some of these things that we should put into consideration when it comes to individualizing the program we have.

For many years, individualization has not been taken seriously, and many have underrated it. Even some experienced psychiatrists do not seem to get it, and many of them may not understand that various patients need different help when it comes to psychotherapy. These people also need various preparedness measures to deal with impending stress due to surgery, and they should be helped differently so that they can effectively deal with allergies, grief, and other issues affecting their lives. But the modern concept does not need to incorporate this hence the reason you see why many meditations have been conditioned to think that there is a particular method of performing psychotherapy that is correct and can be used on various patients and this is the method that they learned from their teachers and mastered it carefully.

Those who try to come up with different concepts both meditation teachers and patients do not succeed in convincing others that there is a need for an individualized program for everyone for it to work well and for the patient to succeed. Many find it easy to believe that there is only one way regardless of what you are dealing with, whether it is meditation, psychotherapy, or other things that need treatment.

They do not want to face the complex situation that every one of different and the best way is to deal with each individual differently, whether this is something complicated or not. However, it would help if you got that we are different individuals with different bodies. When thinking of exercises, do not go for what has been hyped but design your individualized program because this is what can help you get the best results and follow your journey to becoming what you want to become. Are you thinking of changing the movement exercise that you have been doing? If you do not have such an exercise you are doing currently, you can add in your daily program. By looking around, try to know what is appealing to you. You can find an exercise that you are happy with. The kind of exercise you choose should be one that after you are through with the performance, you are left feeling good. If you are good with the popular exercise at the moment, you can go for it, and this could be a sweet coincidence. As you choose the exercise, you need to consider some factors like your current age, the pattern of exercises you were engaged in, and your physique. If you are okay with it, you may decide that you combine several of these exercises and add them to the specific regimen that you already have. You may choose to be jogging every morning, swimming a few laps on two days of the week, and taking a walk on days like Sundays.

As you may have already realized, the subject of the right path for each person lacking has been stressed. Meditation is also not left out, which is one of the best ways to solve various issues for some individuals. It is excellent for many great people around the world to have appreciated many people and it but remember that some people find it to be relevant and not that helpful in their lives. If you are devoted to these meditational exercises and conscientiously perform them for a period of six to eight weeks without seeing results, do not hate yourself because meditation is not your thing. By doing it, your weight cannot become worse, but even if you do not notice the benefits that you were looking for, the advantage that will be there is that you will have undertaken something that you have not done before. At the same time, you will also have engaged your mind to know various things that maybe you did not know about yourself and your body. Even when you find that meditation may not work best when it comes to solving your weight problem, the experience is benefitting, and it will help you learn a lot.

Chapter 9: The Importance of Body Confidence

Self-love is probably the best thing you can accomplish for yourself. Being infatuated with yourself furnishes you with fearlessness, self-esteem and it will by and large help you feel progressively positive. You may likewise find that it is simpler for you to experience passionate feelings for once you have figured out how to cherish yourself first. On the off chance that you can figure out how to adore yourself, you will be a lot more joyful and will figure out how to best deal with yourself paying little respect to the circumstance you are in.

Self-Confidence

Self-confidence is just the demonstration of putting a standard in oneself. Self-confidence as a person's trust in their very own capacities, limits, and decisions, or conviction that the individual in question can effectively confront everyday difficulties and requests. Believing in yourself is one of the most significant ethics to develop so as to make your mind powerful. Fearlessness likewise realizes more bliss. Regularly, when you are sure about your capacities you are more joyful because of your triumphs. When you are resting easy thinking about your abilities, the more stimulated and inspired you are to make a move and accomplish your objectives.

Meditation for Self-Confidence

Sit easily and close your eyes. Count from 1 to 5, concentrating on your breath as you breathe as it were of quiet and unwinding through your nose and breathe out totally through your mouth.

Experience yourself as progressively loose and quiet, prepared to extend your experience of certainty and prosperity right now.

Proceeding to concentrate on your breath, breathing one might say of quiet, unwinding, and breathing out totally.

In the event that you see any strain or snugness in your body, inhale into that piece of your body and as you breathe out experience yourself as progressively loose, quieter.

On the off chance that contemplations enter your psyche, just notice them, and as you breathe out to let them go, proceeding to concentrate on your breath, taking in a more profound feeling of quiet and unwinding and breathing out totally.

Keep on concentrating on our breath as you enable yourself

to completely loosen up your psyche and body, having a feeling of certainty and reestablishment filling your being.

Experience yourself as loose, alert and sure, completely upheld by the seat underneath you. Permitting harmony, satisfaction and certainty to fill your being at this present minute as you currently open yourself to extending your experience of harmony and happiness. And now as you experience yourself as completely present at this time, gradually and easily enable your eyes to open, feeling wide conscious, alert, better than anyone might have expected– completely present at this very moment.

Self-Love

Self-love is not just a condition of feeling better. It is a condition of gratefulness for oneself that develops from activities that help our physical, mental and profound development. Self-love is dynamic; it develops through activities that develop us. When we act in manners that grow self-love in us, we start to acknowledge much better our shortcomings just as our strengths. Self-love is imperative to living great. It impacts who you pick for a mate, the picture you anticipate at work, and how you adapt to the issues throughout your life.

There are such a significant number of methods for rehearsing self-love; it might be by taking a short outing, gifting yourself, beginning a diary or anything that may come as "riches" for you.

Meditation for Self-Love

To start with, make yourself comfortable. Lie on your back with a support under your knees and a collapsed cover behind your head, or sit easily, maybe on a reinforce or a couple collapsed covers. For extra help, do not hesitate to sit against a divider or in a seat.

In the event that you are resting, feel the association between the back of your body and the tangle. On the off chance that you are situated, protract up through your spine, widen through your collarbones, and let your hands lay on your thighs.

When you are settled, close your eyes or mollify your look and tune into your breath. Notice your breath, without attempting to transform it. What's more, see additionally on the off chance that you feel tense or loose, without attempting to change that either.

Breathe in through your nose and afterward breathe out through your mouth. Keep on taking profound, full breaths in through your nose and out through your mouth. As you inhale, become mindful of the condition of your body and the nature of your brain. Where is your body holding pressure?

Do you feel shut off or shut down inwardly? Where is your brain? Is your brain calm or loaded up with fretfulness, antagonism, and uncertainty?

Give your breath a chance to turn out to be progressively smooth and easy and start to take in and out through your nose. Feel the progression of air moving into your lungs and after that pull out into the world. With each breathes out, envision you are discharging any negative considerations that might wait in your brain.

Keep on concentrating on your breath. On each breathe in, think, "I am commendable," and on each breathe out, "I am sufficient." Let each breathe in attract self-esteem and each breathe out discharge what is never again serving you. Take a couple of minutes to inhale and discuss this mantra inside. Notice how you feel as you express these words to yourself.

On the off chance that your mind meanders anytime, realize that it is all right. It is the idea of the brain to meander. Essentially take your consideration back to the breath. Notice how your musings travel in complete disorder, regardless of whether positive or negative and just enable them to pass on by like mists gliding in the sky.

Presently imagine yourself remaining before a mirror and investigate your very own eyes. What do you see? Agony and pity? Love and delight? Lack of bias?

Despite what shows up in the meditation, let yourself know: "I adore you," "You are lovely," and "You are deserving of bliss." Know that what you find in the mirror at this time might be not the same as what you see whenever you look.

Envision since you could inhale into your heart and imagine love spilling out of your hands and into your heart.

Allow this to love warm and saturate you from your heart focus, filling the remainder of your body.

Have a feeling of solace and quiet going up through your chest into your neck and head, out into your shoulders, arms, and hands, and afterward down into your ribs, tummy, pelvis, legs, and feet.

Enable a vibe of warmth to fill you from head to toe. Inhale here and realize that affection is constantly accessible for you when you need it.

When you are prepared, take a couple of all the more profound, careful breaths and after that delicately open your eyes. Sit for a couple of minutes to recognize the one of a kind encounter you had during this meditation.

Chapter 10: Hypnosis Myths

It is common to misjudge the topic of hypnotism. That is why myths and half-truths abound about this matter.

Myth: You won't recall that anything that happened when you were mesmerized when you wake up from a trance.

While amnesia may occur in uncommon cases, during mesmerizing, people more often than not recollect everything that unfolded. Mesmerizing, be that as it may, can have a significant memory impact. Posthypnotic amnesia may make an individual overlook a portion of the stuff that occurred previously or during spellbinding. This effect, be that as it may, is typically confined and impermanent.

Myth: Hypnosis can help people to recall the exact date of wrongdoing they have been seeing.

While spellbinding can be utilized to improve memory, the effects in well-known media have been significantly misrepresented. Research has discovered that trance doesn't bring about noteworthy memory improvement or precision, and entrancing may, in reality, lead to false or misshaped recollections.

Myth: You can be spellbound against your will

Spellbinding needs willful patient investment regardless of stories about people being mesmerized without their authorization.

Myth: While you are under a trance, the trance specialist has full power over your conduct.

While individuals frequently feel that their activities under trance appear to happen without their will's impact, a trance specialist can't make you act against your wants.

Myth: You might be super-solid, brisk, or physically gifted with trance.

While mesmerizing can be utilized for execution upgrade, it can't make people more grounded or more athletic than their physical abilities.

Myth: Everyone can be entranced

It is beyond the realm of imagination to expect to entrance everybody. One research shows that it is amazingly hypnotizable around 10 percent of the populace. While it might be attainable to spellbind the rest of the masses, they are more reluctant to be open to the activity.

Myth: You are responsible for your body during trance

Despite what you see with stage trance, you will remain aware of what you are doing and what you are being mentioned. On the off chance that you would prefer not to do anything under mesmerizing, you're not going to do it.

Myth: Hypnosis is equivalent to rest.

You may look like resting, yet during mesmerizing, you are alert. You're just in a condition of profound unwinding. Your muscles will get limp, your breathing rate will back off, and you may get sleepy.

Myth: When mesmerized, individuals can't lie,

Sleep induction isn't a truth serum in the real world. Even though during subliminal therapy, you are progressively open to a recommendation, regardless; you have through and through freedom and good judgment. Nobody can make you state anything you would prefer not to say—lie or not.

Myth: Many cell phone applications and web recordings empower self-trance, yet they are likely inadequate.

Analysts in a 2013 survey found that such instruments are not ordinarily created by an authorized trance inducer or mesmerizing association. Specialists and subliminal specialists consequently prescribe against utilizing these.

Most likely, a myth: entrancing can help you "find" lost recollections.

Even though recollections can be recouped during mesmerizing, while in a daze like a state, you might be bound to create false recollections. Along these lines, numerous trance specialists remain distrustful about memory recovery utilizing spellbinding.

The primary concern entrancing holds the stage execution

generalizations, alongside clacking chickens and influential artists.

Trance, be that as it may, is a genuine remedial instrument and can be utilized for a few conditions as an elective restorative treatment. This includes the administration of a sleeping disorder, grief, and agony.

You utilize a trance specialist or subliminal specialist authorized to confide in the technique for guided trance. An organized arrangement will be made to help you accomplish your individual goals.

Conclusion

Let's look back at our progress and then paying it forward to others. Continue eating better all day. You'll feel better, look better, achieve your goals, and have a better quality of life. Assuming you've read and understood all the content here, chances are that you've realized your habits and applying core solutions to overcoming obstacles while holding yourself accountable, you have Paid attention to yourself, your purpose, unique talents, and dreams. By automating your food and water, cutting out unhealthy sugar, alcohol and white carbs, adding protein, Greek yogurt or other probiotics, produce and healthy fats.

Choose to continue with the same eating habit all your life. Focus on a healthy weight; stay with silence. Visualize your step and take steps that are going to get you to where you want to be. If you destabilize procrastination, stress and comfort zone, you will go farther at a fast pace. Organize your kitchen and automate your food. Be a reader; Read positive affirmations aloud every day. Pursue your goals, including your fitness and health goals that will utilize your talents and passions and keep you on the healthy-fit journey. Rest on weekends and follow the process again.

Focus on your activities, journalize your progress, thoughts, and move on. Record your success, nature; they will guide you in thinking and solving stress, among other problems. You will make not only an impact on yourself but also the people around you. Make use of productivity apps on the internet to guide you through.

While writing your journal, consider how you've grown physically, mentally, spiritually, and emotionally or socially. Think about how one area has positively affected other areas. If some things haven't worked out for you, spend some time forgiving other people, forgiving yourself so you can move on. Giving makes living worthwhile.

Albert Einstein believed that a life shared with others is worthy. We have people out there who need you, remember not to hoard your successes. Share your success. Share your new-found recipes, your attitude, and your habits. Share what you have learned with others. In all your undertakings, know that you can't change other people but yourself, therefore, be mindful. Reflect on your changes and put yourself on the back today and every day. Be grateful and live your life as a champion.

Make it a reality on your mind, the fact that the journey to a healthy life and weight loss is long and has many challenges. Pieces of Stuff we consider more important in life require our full cooperation towards them. Just because you are facing problems in your Wight loss journey, it does not mean that you should stop, instead show and prove the whole world how good your ability to handle constant challenges is—training your brain to know that eating healthy food together with functional exercises can work miracles. Make it your choice and not something you are forced to do by a third party. Always tell yourself that weight loss is a long process and not an event. Take every day of your days to celebrate your achievements because these achievements are what piles up to a massive victory. Make a list of stuff you would like to change when you get healthy they may be Small size-clothes, being able to accumulate enough energy, participating in your most loved sports you have been admiring for a more extended period, feeling self-assured. Make these tips your number one source of empowerment; you will end up completing your 30 days even without noticing.

You have made it, or you are about to make it. The journey has been unbelievable. And by now, you must be having a story to tell. Concentrate on finishing strongly. Keep up the excellent eating design you have adopted. Remember, you are not working on temporary changes but long-term goals. Therefore, lifestyle changes should not be stopped when the weight is lost. Remind yourself always of essential habits that are easier to follow daily. They include trusting yourself and the process by acknowledging that the real change lies in your hands. Stop complacency, arise, and walk around for at least thirty minutes away. Your breakfast is the most important meal you deserve. Eat your breakfast like a queen. For each diet, you take, add a few proteins and natural fats. Let hunger not kill you, eat more, but just what is recommended, bring snacks and other meals 3 or 5 times a day. Have more veggies and fruits like 5-6 rounds in 24 hours. Almost 90% of Americans do not receive enough vegetables and fruits to their satisfaction. Remember, Apple will not make you grow fat. Substitute salt. You will be shocked by the sweet taste of food once you stop consuming salt. Regain your original feeling, you will differentiate natural flavorings from artificial flavors. Just brainstorm how those older adults managed to eat their food without salt or modern-day characters. Characters are not suitable for your health. Drink a lot of water in a day. Let water be your number one drink. Avoid soft drinks and other energy drinks, and they are slowly killing you. Drink a lot of water in the morning after getting out of your bed. Your body will be fresh from morning to evening. Have a journal and be realistic with it. Take charge of what you write and be responsible.

CPSIA information can be obtained
at www.ICGtesting.com
Printed in the USA
BVHW050449060321
601819BV00002B/46